Table of Contents

M000082411

**My weight loss journey:
How I lost 44 pounds and never gained them back using a
plant based diet.**

by Andreas Michaelides

My weight loss journey: How I lost 44 pounds and never gained them back using a plant based diet.

ISBN: 978-9963-2285-0-8 print version
Cyprus Library.
www.cypruslibrary.gov.cy

About the Author.

Andreas was born in Athens, the city that gave birth to Democracy, in Greece, the country that taught to the world how to live, think, and have fun. He grew up on the beautiful island of Cyprus.

With both of his parent's bibliophiles (and his father a high school teacher), Andreas grew up with love and appreciation for literature. In addition to the books he borrowed from the school library, a stack of encyclopedias taught him about the world. A history lover from age 13, he devoured the memoirs of Winston Churchill and Charles de Gaul, and by age 17, he had read all of Julius Vern's books.

After serving his country for 26 months immediately after finishing high school, Andreas studied in Patra, Greece to become a computer engineer. With his Master of Computer Engineering and Informatics, he began working in the Informatics Department of the local university hospital and started reading again with a vengeance.

In 2004, Andreas authored his first book, a historical novel that has not yet seen the light of publication. Leaving it unpublished made him feel like a failure, but a lot has changed since then. Eleven years later, he has successfully quit smoking and has been smoke-free for the past seven years. He has also started running again and managed to lose 26 kg (57 lbs).

Andreas has run three marathons, as well as many half-marathons and other shorter races. His love for running is what renewed him and actually saved his life.

Multiple medical problems pushed Andreas to research and experiment with a plant-based diet; since 2013 he is following a whole plant based diet.

In addition to running, Andreas enjoys hiking, cycling, playing basketball, camping, photography, and going out with friends and family and having fun.

You can follow the writer at his web page www.thirsty4health.com.

Prologue

Hello, my name is Andreas. On the 8th of September 2016, I turned forty-two years old! Wow, I remember when I was twenty years old, just after my twenty-six-month military service ended, that I thought that until I reached forty, I would have had twenty whole years ahead of me to enjoy life and do whatever I was dreaming of or whatever I thought was a good life back then.

I would have had time to go to the university to follow my chosen passion which was computer engineering, I would have found a great job that pays good money and traveled the entire world with a beautiful, sexy lady by my side.

I would have met and fallen in love with the perfect woman, bought the perfect car, and built the perfect house so I can create my perfect family with lots of kids. But not because I wanted those things, but maybe because the Cypriot society has idealized such a lifestyle, making you think that this is the right road for you.

So I felt compelled to do all of these things (studying, falling in love, getting married, having kids, building a house, having a car, a good job and traveling) because as I was getting closer and closer to my forties, my chances to accomplish all these wonderful daydreams were diminishing, day in and day out.
Tick tock, the years were passing, and forty was not as far anymore as it used to be.

On the back of the mind of a twenty-year-old, forty is always something distant and way too far into the future. Also, forty for me always brought to mind an image of a married man with three kids, big belly, bald head, with a cigarette in one hand and a beer in the other, eating Souvlaki with his family in a Greek tavern on the weekends.

That is how many 40-year-olds and older are in the country I live in, Cyprus, this beautiful Greek island that has the misfortune of being situated in an excellent, and thus desirable, political, economic, geographical, and strategic place in the eastern part of the Mediterranean Sea.

Most men around this age and older here in Cyprus are out of shape, have high blood pressure, high cholesterol, and lots of them have diabetes II or are heading that way. Many of them also have male potency problems.

They mostly suffer from kidney stones, arthritis, heart conditions like angina, and blocked heart arteries, while there is also a significant number of them with prostate cancer, colon cancer, stomach ulcer, and a series of other so-called western chronic diseases.

You can imagine now why a twenty-year-old man didn't want to turn forty that fast; because, to my then ignorant mind, all the conditions and illnesses I described seemed to be unavoidable.

Sadly, there are people in this country, and in the entire planet, of course, that still assume that when you turn forty, your life starts to go downhill as far as your health is concerned. I mean most people now die around sixty to eighty years old, so forty is like half your life on this planet, right? Well, wrong!

I am here to tell you that all that is misinformation about the true potential of the human body and that the human lifespan is three times forty! Yes, you read it right, we have the biological capacity to reach one hundred and twenty years of age easily with a proper plant-based diet and a sensible exercise regime. We can have long and quality years on this beautiful green-blue planet, without drugs and surgeries or any other gadget or medieval construction that the doctors and the pharmaceutical companies invent just to take your hard-earned money out of your pockets.

If you are reading this book, it is probably because you want to lose weight and most important never to gain it back. You are struggling for years with various diets to lose weight, but it always comes back, right?

I am sure you spent or are spending a lot of money buying videotapes or DVDs or books that claim they can make you lose weight fast and easy.

Well, let me tell you something, my dear reader. Basically, I can totally feel you because ten years ago, I used to be that person too. Like you today, I was struggling with obesity and weight problems. I thought that by following a certain diet or applying myself to an exercise regime for a specific timeframe, I would lose my kilos fast and easy. Here are those two words again: fast and easy.

These two words actually do magic; if you put them in the same sentence, you can sell a property on the moon and get away with it. Don't you believe me? Here are a few examples:

"Buy this amazing abs machine and get awesome abs in just 2 weeks (fast) and with no effort at all (easy)." Another example, "Buy this incredible green tea and lose 10 kilos in 2 weeks (fast) and in the comfort of your home (easy)."

Shall I mention another example? No, I don't think you need one. I am sure you got the point just as I'm sure that you have tried various useless diets that ended up making you gain more weight, making you feel worse about yourself, and you may have spent a lot of money on workout machines that fail to do what they promise.

A lot of you spend a fortune on magical supplements and other pills that are supposed to give you the slender figure you desire, and of course, FAST and EASY. Well, I am here to tell you this, and with this, I will end my prologue and then prove my point in the rest of the book.

No diet, exercise machine, magic tea or pill is going to make you lose weight fast and easy; this is impossible. Surely, you will see some weight loss, which is mostly water anyway, but it only lasts as long as you do the diet, which for its most part is unhealthy in the first place.

If you want to lose weight and never gain it back, please read my story and see how I did it.

With my story and the philosophy that comes out of it, as far as weight loss is concerned, you are going to lose weight healthily, and you will not gain it back. You will lose it not FAST, but gradually. It is not going to be EASY; it is going to be an adventure. So if you think you have the patience and a little bit of an adventure bug in your life, please continue reading.

The Digestive System

It took me a while to realize that my daily practice of consuming non-nutritious food, as well as my nicotine addiction, overloaded my digestive system, which then caused a chain reaction to multiple health problems.

The human body is an incredible, unique biological machine that has many subsystems, including the digestive system. Upon learning more about how the human body works, I had an epiphany: the health problems that I was suffering from were caused by the foods I ate. Something as simple and easily changeable as a poor diet had led to numerous health issues, including heartburn, stomach ulcers, hemorrhoids, constipation, and bloated intestines. You see, the rest of my body's systems were in bad shape and malfunctioning because they all depended on my digestive system to get the nutrients they needed.

Each person's wake-up call is different; mine was struggling with health problems related to my digestive system. After that revelation, I started learning more about that matter, as knowledge is power. Knowing how my body works has allowed me to get to the path I am now on, which includes following a healthy diet plan.

My new diet is radically different from that old one of excessive quantities of meat, dairy, and few (if any) veggies. I now follow a plant-based diet that is 80% raw and 20% cooked. I always question and experiment with it, and nutrition has now been a subject about which I will never get tired of learning.

Eat Like a Chef

I never used to chew my food; I would gulp it, like a lion, sending big chunks of food into my stomach, without it being correctly processed by the saliva in my mouth, which forced my stomach to work harder and longer, and sometimes gave me indigestion. I learned this bad habit from my mother who also gulps her food. However, I now consciously train myself to chew every mouthful thoroughly before I swallow. You don't have to count the number of chews per bite; just eat at a slower pace and be patient rather than hurrying through your meal. You will enjoy your meal more and feel more satisfied if you eat in that manner.

When you sit down to eat, make sure there are no distractions. Turn off your TV and radio, and don't play with your mobile phone or tablet while at the table eating. Eat your food as if you are a chef who is discovering every single ingredient in a new entrée by taste alone; feel it, rather than devouring and hardly noticing how delicious your meal is. These tips will also discourage you from mindlessly eating way too much; simply by slowing down, you will enjoy your food more and be more aware of how much your body needs before you are no longer hungry.

The time you eat must be sacred; it should not be merely nourishment for your body, but also for your spirit. Eating in a quiet environment with no other distractions is a good start. When you eat, you should only hear the light sound of the silverware lightly touching the plate.

Do not eat for the sake of becoming full, but for the benefit of no longer being hungry; in some cultures, it is considered healthy to eat until you are about 70% full, rather than eating until you feel as though you just finished Thanksgiving dinner.

Do Your Research

I recommend studying more how the body works, what you can do to improve your diet, and how important vegetables are to your overall health. Check that every health article you are reading is written by someone with valid credentials, such as a nutritionist, doctor, or expert in the field of health. If they are not an expert themselves, you can always check their article's sources to verify their claims.

Read recent articles about health topics, not articles or books that are five or more years old, as research results are regularly updated to include significant new findings. Outdated studies will provide outdated knowledge. Also, avoid fad diet books, which will only discourage you from pursuing good health due to their lack of substantive research-based information.

Read scientific papers from writers who do not have a conflict of interest. For example, if you are reading an article that says eggs are good for your health, but you notice that the researcher got a significant grant from the egg industry, then you know that he or she is biased. It's logical, of course; the writer would present a paper that favors egg consumption if they are being paid by the egg industry.

Read scientific papers that are sponsored by independent organizations, whose funding does not come from the meat or dairy industry, and so on. They are out there; you just need to search a little to find the subject you're looking.

Go For Regular Health Checkups

Medical problems will always arise in our life, and one of the most important health habits that we should have is to always go for regular checkups with our doctor. Never play the doctor yourself, reading about your symptoms online. They can be too broad to provide an accurate diagnosis or can lead you to believe you have a serious illness because the symptoms sometimes can coincide.

While your doctor can give you advice on nutrition, it is better to seek advice from a licensed nutritionist who is better trained and educated; on average, doctors have received only three hours of nutritional education in school.

Vital Information

You can find the above excerpt in my first book, Thirsty for Health. It pinpoints critical information so you can lose the weight you desire safely and healthily and never get it back in the long run.

Since you chose to read this book, it means that either you started adopting a plant-based diet, or you are just trying to find out more about the topic, which is a good thing. I assume that I am speaking to an individual who started questioning everything about what is nutritionally right or wrong—and, trust me, there are a lot of wrongs nutrition-wise on this planet.

There are thousands of scientific articles out there that prove beyond a reasonable doubt that as one's diet focuses on plants, he or she deals with fewer diseases and illnesses, and the overall quality of life is much better than that of the omnivores.

I can't stress this enough, a plant-based diet and especially one with whole food is the diet you should adopt if you want to be able to lose the excess weight safely, healthily, and once and for all.

If you do not believe me—and I hope so; I don't want believers, I want questioners, I want you to be a soldier of knowledge and research—go out there and search, and when you are done, do some more search! NEVER STOP SEARCHING AND RESEARCHING, especially such a sensitive matter as what you put in your mouth day in and day out.

Now some of you may say: "Andreas, don't be mean, I can't just stop eating my meat or have my warm glass of milk before I go to bed or this or that…" Hey, I understand you, I am not one of those crazy "vegan" activists that grab people by the neck because they still eat meat or consume dairy products or still eat seafood or fish. I am not. I understand you because I used to be one of you until 2013. I used to eat lots of meat so, as a former omnivore, I can advise you on a subtle start.

Start with something simple

Yes, I did say that losing weight is not achieved fast and easy but to get there, you need to make baby steps, and guess what? Baby steps *are* easy.

For a start, do not change your current diet; what I ask of you is to add one to two fruits daily and have a green salad with your lunch or dinner three times a week. Try that for a month or ten days or even a week. You will see that you will feel better because the fruits and the salad contain fiber, and they are also full of antioxidants, vitamins, minerals, and phytonutrients that will make your body feel better.

I am sure that by adding a little more fibrous food to your diet, like fruits and vegetables, you will eat less non-fibrous food like meat, dairy, and so on because fiber keeps you full for longer periods.

I mean, think about it, how hard is it to eat two apples at work? Or while going to work, either on a bus, a train or metro? And if not apples, then two oranges, two pears, and so on. You can have them as a late snack 30 to 45 minutes before you go to bed. Have a banana, for example, which also help you sleep and have calming properties.

You just wash them and eat them, you don't even have to peel them or cut them, eat them as they are meant to be eaten.

How hard is to make a green salad with maybe three or four ingredients? You can have some lettuce, tomato, cucumber, and some white onion. Furthermore, you can add some nuts, like walnuts or pumpkin nuts and so on. The internet is full of vegetarian and vegan recipes to get inspiration from.

You can even prepare a small salad at night, and you can have it at work the next day. The possibilities are endless, and it is in your hand to make it happen.

Try and just do this for starters, just add one to two fruits in your diet daily—when and how you eat them is your decision. Also, try having vegetables three times a week, either for lunch or dinner, or just a snack of green salad with three to four ingredients in it. Try this for a month, and you will see a change in your health, I am sure.

So Many Challenges Out There

If you feel psychologically stronger and decisive to eliminate meat and dairy for the most part, then there are various plant-based diets that you can adopt. A lot of webpages out there offer help with that. It's only a matter of you using the internet not just for entertainment but also to research something that will have an immediate impact on your health and your quality of life.

Here is a list of a few plant-based (vegan) challenges:

http://veganeasy.org/vegan-easy-challenge
http://www.bodyrock.tv/food/one-month-vegan-challenge/
http://7dayvegan.com/
http://www.govegan.org.uk/
http://veganyogalife.com/why-i-am-going-vegan-at-least-for-a-month/

I do not earn any money by suggesting these links to you, nor am I an affiliate of these sites, just to make things clear. I am just referring them to you to see how easy it is to find this kind of information.

Another thing that is going to help you with your weight loss and also with your general health is chewing slowly and making sure your food has a creamy texture before you swallow it. The smaller the size of food going into the stomach, the easier it is for the stomach to make the digestion.

Additionally, make sure you eat in an environment that promotes tranquility and a sense of relaxation. You may not see it now, but a relaxed mind leads to a relaxed body, which plays a significant role in the nutrient absorption.

Lastly, I would like to give you a link of one of the people that opened my eyes regarding nutrition and, in a sense, saved my life.
GO right now and visit the site www.nutritionfacts.org and sign up. Registering at this good Doc's site is going to be the best thing you ever did nutrition-wise.

The site is run by Dr. Michael Greger, MD who's been a plant-based and whole-food advocate for years now. The site is entirely based on donations and is economically backed by the Canadian philanthropist, Jesse Rasch, and his wife, Julie. This site cares about the people and provides them with the real science that is free from political, economic or personal interests. He also recently published an excellent book called How Not To Die which I urge you to buy without hesitation.

The next chapter tells my story, which is also included in my first book, Thirsty for Health. I am sure that you will relate to my story and that, after reading it, you will connect with me even more. It's here also to show you that I am not a superman for accomplishing the loss of all those pounds (44 to be exact); I am just a regular man who saw the light regarding nutrition and applied himself not only to achieve this incredible weight loss but also to maintain the new weight till today.

Now that I am writing these words, I am 74 kg (about 160 pounds) and 1.74 m tall (5'.9"), and I have been like this since 2013.

Here's my story, ladies and gentlemen. Enjoy!

My weight Problem

While growing up, I was always thin. As a family, we were not fat, and my relatives were neither overweight nor obese.

I was an athlete during high school, so I was pretty lean. When I joined the Army, I weighed 60 kg (132 lbs.), and when I left it, I was at 82 kg (180.5 lbs.)! That's when I realized I was overweight for the first time in my life. Army food—which, by my standards today, was too fatty—plus all the junk food I was eating contributed to me gaining 22 kg (48.5 lbs.). At some point, the exercises that had been keeping me in relatively good shape began to become rarer and rarer, which slowed down my metabolism and also contributed to my accumulation of all the excess weight.

Back then, I had no idea which factors determine one's weight. I now know that these factors are our genes (meaning our DNA), our metabolic rate (the rate we burn calories to produce energy), our eating patterns, and our exercise regimen.

I knew I had good genes, as my parents and my grandparents had all been thin while they were young, so I had that in my favor. So if my genes weren't to blame, why had I become overweight? We are not slaves of our genes, as many people think. Some people see a fat person and immediately assume he or she must be genetically prone to being fat.

The fact is that genes are only one's starting point; they are the "default" that can be overcome with a proper diet and exercise program. My research into this issue showed that genes determine only a 3-5 percent of one's weight; the remaining 95-97 percent is controlled by you and your lifestyle choices. Our fate is not determined solely by genes; one's lifestyle makes much more of a difference than genetics.

While I couldn't change my genes, which weren't that bad anyway, I could change my metabolic rate by improving my eating habits and following a better exercise routine. I knew I couldn't make excuses anymore. I wasn't fat because of bad genes; I was fat because I overate the wrong foods and didn't exercise enough.

The cause of the obesity epidemic in western societies and organizations that adopt the standard American diet is partly due to the agricultural and technological innovations of the past few centuries, which have made food very easy to acquire and have vastly reduced the need for physical labor. In the modern world, most of us no longer need our evolutionary adaptations such as storing fat for times of famine or having a body suitable for acquiring our food under harsh conditions (such as in the times of many peasants working the fields or hunters stalking their prey over long distances).

While I was in the army, I relied on genetics, believing I would never get fat because my parents were not obese either. But by not getting enough exercise, my metabolic rate slowed, and my diet consisted almost entirely of junk food and the army's fatty food.

Primarily, I was consuming more calories than I was burning, and the excess calories were stored in my body as fat; it accumulated to a 22-kg (48.5 lbs.) gain in twenty-six months.

After the army, I went to study in Greece. I lost approximately 25 kg (55 lbs.), and I was between 55 and 60 kg (121 and 132 pounds) until the age of thirty-one.

When I returned to Cyprus in 2005, I was around 60-65 kg (132-143 pounds). I started eating three times a day because I got much higher quality food than I used to (since my mother was cooking for me, it was so good so I would eat more.)

From 2005 until 2009, I gained another 20 kg (44lbs). I was hovering between 80 and 85kg (176 and 187 lbs.). Back then, I still had my faith that my good genes alone would save me from becoming overweight, and the only difference in my diet was I stopped drinking coffee and caffeinated sodas because I was diagnosed with ulcers.

Another reason for my weight gain was that none of my three jobs were active ones; I am a computer engineer, so my work involves sitting in front of a computer eight to twelve hours a day, so I was living a sedentary lifestyle, as I never went to the gym or exercised. Making matters worse, I would eat chips, chocolates, and any other processed junk food full of too much salt, fat, and sugar; an excess of calories contributed to my weight gain.

In 2009, I quit smoking. I weighed between 82 and 84 kg (181 and 185 lbs.). Anyone who has tried to quit smoking knows about the subconscious need and tendency that urge you to do something with your hands and your mouth. The course of action of smoking is another part of the addiction: getting out a cigarette, putting it in your mouth, lighting it, bringing down the lighter, and most of all, holding the cigarette in your mouth—you have trained yourself to psychologically connect these actions with the initial rush of nicotine.

So since I quit smoking, I had the subconscious tendency to keep my hands and mouth occupied; this led me to eat and drink all the time—mostly junk food like chips, chocolates, iced tea, and processed juices.

When 2010 arrived, exactly one year after I stopped smoking, I realized that I had gained another 10 kg (22 lbs.). At thirty-six years old, I weighed between 92 and 94 kg (203 and 207 pounds) and stood 1.74 m tall (5'9''). If I didn't change my lifestyle, I would be obese in a year, and severe problems would start to emerge. I was knocking on obesity's door.

This meant I was putting myself at risk for the following diseases and health problems:

- Heart problems
- High blood pressure

- Elevated LDL("bad") cholesterol and triglycerides
- Lowered HDL("good") cholesterol abnormal heartbeat
- Angina
- Heart disease
- Heart attack
- Heart failure
- Coronary artery disease
- Stroke
- Prostate cancer
- Gallbladder
- Cancer colorectal
- Cancer
- Cancer kidney
- Cancer
- Breast cancer (yes, some men have breast cancer)
- Liver problems
- Enlarged liver
- Cirrhosis of the liver
- Fatty liver
- Breathing problems
- Sleep apnea (snoring, difficulty in breathing while asleep)
- Asthma
- Other medical problems
- Type II diabetes
- GERD (acid reflux)
- Arthritis
- Memory & learning problems

At just thirty-six years old, I was a candidate for anyone of those health problems. When I saw the number on the scale, I didn't believe it; I assumed that the machine was broken. It took me a few days to realize how fat I was.

I would see myself in the mirror every day in the morning when I was washing my face, shaving, or drying off after a shower; I could see my shape, but I wasn't really looking at myself. Instead, I was relying on how I remembered myself as a strong, lean teenager twenty years ago! I honestly thought I was thin until a few days after I got on that scale.

A colleague from work once said that when you look at your face in the mirror, you don't acknowledge that you are getting older. You realize it when others say it to you, or something happens that makes you look yourself as you are—then maybe you will be able to escape that "Matrix" virtual life you've convinced yourself you live.

After I got the results of my blood tests, which verified how unhealthy of a condition my body was in, I got the red pill (as Neo did in the movie). I started to accept the painful reality that I was fat. I decided that I had to do something so that every time I looked at myself in the mirror, I would see a healthy, lean individual, not an overweight and out-of-shape man.

The only reason that I started to walk and then run was out of sheer vanity. I wanted to look good, and I saw exercise as a temporary chore that I would keep it up only until I became thin again. Once that happened, I would stop activity altogether.

I had no idea that running would become a permanent part of a new lifestyle for me.

Although I started to exercise for the wrong reasons—meaning my motives were unrelated to health—I now run for my health and have embraced regular exercise as my way of living. If I don't exercise at least every other day now, I get sick to my stomach and feel depressed.

When I started running and walking, I kept a calendar in Excel sheet to track my progress, which helped me to overcome the threat of lapsing back into my sedentary lifestyle.

There were times when I was so tired and fatigued that I seriously questioned why I was torturing myself with running. I could be home sitting on my couch in front of my big-screen TV devouring some tasty chips and a nice cup of iced tea, watching an action movie in which all of the exercises are done by actors.

Unlike when I quit smoking, during which I had my father's support as we both quit smoking together, I was alone in my effort of losing weight. I had no company while faced with my challenge of weight loss. I ran alone: whenever I would go running on the track, there was nobody else there. Of a village of eight hundred people, nobody went running at the same time as me. Sometimes a couple of people went there to walk, but for a short period, and they were older than me—besides, they were walking, not running. So being lonely in my endeavor sometimes made me feel discouraged, and I questioned my actions.

Frustration at not increasing my mileage or losing weight rapidly enough was the third issue; I got angry about this often, especially during the first two months.

Four of the main factors that push people to lapse back into their previous situation are H.A.L.T. (Hungry, Angry, Lonely, and Tired). I had three of these factors, but I was not hungry because I ate anything I wanted (I was relying on exercise alone to shed weight, ignoring the importance of a healthy diet).

I had small lapses, such as times when I didn't feel like going out at 8 p.m. to run, and sometimes I would stay in bed dozing or watching a movie. My diary helped me because whenever I was angry or tired or feeling alone, I would open it up and see my progress from where I had started to where I was now. I could see the transformation of a couch potato into an active person, which brought me feelings of satisfaction, pride, and happiness. Those positive emotions helped me to forget my loneliness, my tiredness, and my anger immediately, and I would refocus on my goal of becoming a lean, sinewy running machine and losing weight along the way. It was my diary that helped me to get through some difficult moments when I was on the edge of quitting; I heartily recommend keeping one for any task you wish to fulfill.

The first entry in my running diary says that on April 26th, 2010, I ran 900 meters and burned 56.25 calories.

Back then, I didn't have a device to measure the number of calories I was burning, so I was using equations that were based on my weight, height, etc., which I incorporated into the Excel sheet. Tracking this helped me to be more involved in the whole endeavor; I couldn't wait to go outside to walk and run so I would have some data to input into the Excel sheet so I could see my results and analyze the time spent and calories burned. Being able to set my progress down and see it in actual numbers encouraged me to keep up my exercise routine.

When searching to see how far from the average weight I was (so I would know how much weight I should lose), I discovered the BMI (Body Mass Index), which is a standard that determines a healthy weight. One's BMI is calculated by dividing one's weight in kg by our height in meters raised to the second power. In 2010, I was 94 kg and 1.74 meters tall; the equation to find my BMI is $94 / (1.74)^2$, which equals $94/3.0276$, which gives us the result 31.05.

According to the BMI chart, I was in the first stages of obesity. Now that I am 74 kg, the equation becomes $74 / (1.74)^2$, which equals $74/3.0276$, which gives us the result 24.45—a vast improvement. However, I am on the upper limit of normal, which means I need to lose a few more kilos to situate myself in the middle of the standard zone, which will be more desirable.

Although knowing one's BMI is helpful, he or she should not depend on it exclusively; many other factors define and determine one's healthy weight. For example, if I started bodybuilding, then I might gain weight and reach 80 kg. Using the math above, that would give me a BMI of 26.43, which would bring me back to the overweight zone. However, the truth would be that I would have a higher ratio of muscle to fat, so although I would be classed as "overweight," the truth is I would still be healthy.

Your body type, which is heavily dependent on your genes, is another factor to consider. There are three basic body types (and there are combinations of them). These body types influence, to some degree, our response to diets and training. It is paramount to identify and understand your body type so that you can efficiently and correctly plan your muscle building training and diet program—or any other athletic endeavor you want to pursue.

The first body type is the ectomorph. It is your everyday, typical skinny man. Their physical build is light, with a petite frame and lean muscles. Usually, people in this category have thin, elongated limbs with fibrous muscles, and their shoulders tend towards a compact structure and small width.

The second body type is the mesomorph. People with this body type have a large frame, moderately large muscles, and a natural athletic appearance. Mesomorph is the ideal body type for bodybuilders. They gain weight quite easy and can also find it quite easy to lose weight. They are naturally strong, which is the perfect basis to build muscles.

The third body type is the endomorph. People with this body type have a robust and soft body. They are weight-gainers, meaning they gain weight very quickly. They are usually shorter in height compared with the two previous body types and usually have thick arms and legs. Their muscles are strong, especially their upper legs. They do well with leg exercises, especially squats.

As there are combinations of the three main body types, some people could be ectomorph-mesomorph—that's me, by the way—or mesomorph-endomorph. Once you understand how your body works, it becomes easier to find the tools to make your health and fitness goals happen (even if they are based on vanity); all you need is determination.

I knew that if I were serious about losing weight, I would need to find a training and diet program that would fit my particular body type combination. I classed myself as an ectomorph-mesomorph because I gain weight easily, but I also lose weight quickly; I had a yo-yo weight—on-off 20 kg (44 lbs.)—at least twice in my life. The ectomorph part of me is my chest and shoulders, which are thin and not wide enough; I don't get much weight there.

Although I never expected to drag myself out of the house and go for a run, after I finished those first three rounds at the high school track in my village, everything changed. I was so exhausted—which was an indicator of how poor my fitness was—but after all the discomfort, itching, and rashes in various places due to friction from excess fat, for the first time, I felt renewed. Memories of running and winning first place in high school reminded me of how I used to be, compared to how I was after those three laps around the track.

It made my eyes water; I was alone in the middle of that track under an April sky full of stars when tears of mixed feelings started pouring down. Emotionally and psychologically, it was a turning point for me, and it also made me even more determined to become that lean, mean running machine I used to be. It was right there, in that single moment that I saw the path I had to follow.

I continued to run and walk day by day, gradually increasing my running and walking distance. At first, I was walking; then, walking and running; and finally, only running.
I was convinced that by just running, I would lose the extra weight I was carrying. I was, of course, dead wrong.

During the first six months of running and walking, I lost a lot of weight (about 14 kg/31 lbs.). I was jubilant at achieving it. So, seeing my weight loss from running reinforced my preexisting false belief that I could get rid of all the extra weight only by running.

Almost six months after I started exercising, on October 10th, 2010, I ran my first half-marathon! I couldn't believe it; I think it took me a few days to realize I had accomplished it.

I had started off as a depressed, anxious, lethargic fat guy with low self-esteem and no interest in exercise, and just six months later, I had run my first half-marathon—that's 21 km, people! It was the farthest distance I had ever run at the time—by then, my record was 6 km from my high school days—and I did it in 2 hours and 18 minutes.

One week after I ran my first half-marathon, I went to Bucharest, Romania, and ran the half-marathon there in 2 hours and 9 minutes. My time was faster by 9 minutes—I know the course was not the same, but both races were flat and about the same altitude—which made me euphoric and boosted my confidence.

Unfortunately, though, it derailed me from my basic goal, to lose my extra weight. It awakened my competitive bug, which was asleep since my running years in high school. Firstly, I wanted to be the best me I could be, and secondly to be better than others. In every other future half-marathon, I wanted my performance to be better than the previous one, and to see how much faster I could go.

Through my desire to become more competitive, I discovered that food and athletics are connected. With each book I read, along with experimentation through trial-and-error, I managed to be where I am today.

For the next two years, I would steadily weigh 78 kg (172 lbs.), and my weight would not go down. It was frustrating. No matter how much running I did, my weight remained unchanged, even though I was running long distances—in 2011, I ran a total of 2,479 km (1,540 miles)!

From 2011 until 2013, I constantly wondered why I didn't lose any more weight; in my mind, I was doing everything right and going by the book.

Had I not aimed to better my athletic performance in half-marathon races, then my only issue would have been the weight loss of the remaining 6 to 8 kilos (13 to 18 lbs.). I researched what to eat to be faster and stronger, rather than researching what to eat to lose weight; these two concepts do not go together. You either set up your goal to lose weight or to excel in athletic performance; nutritionally and athletically, you cannot achieve both at the same time—I tried it, and I failed miserably.

As far as nutrition is concerned, both avenues helped me tremendously. I know now not to try to accomplish two things at the same time. If I want to run a race, my goal is an athletic performance improvement. The distance doesn't matter now, as I have accepted the fact that I will not lose any weight by racing. To lose weight, I need to use a different plan.

Complete New Person

Wow, right? Sometimes I read this story, and I feel so disconnected that I wonder if someone else wrote it.

I am an entirely new person now, but every time I want to start eating junk food again or skip a running session, I always have a copy of this story on my desk at home or work or even in my car. I have it on my mobile phone, and whenever I feel weak or forget why I am doing what I am doing, I read this story, and everything becomes clear again.

Again, I am not asking you to become a plant-based eater overnight, but if you want to be able to shed the weight off and never get it back, you must set it as a long-term goal to become a plant-based eater. At least minimize as much as you can the animal consumption to the level you feel comfortable with. Don't just do it because you HAVE TO DO IT. The moment you feel like that, then you lost the game and the opportunity to become something better health-wise and nutrition-wise. Remember, *baby steps*.

So, as you read in my story, I was struggling to lose weight only through regular exercising, and my exercise was, and still is, running.

Secret Of Weight Loss

The secret to weight loss and maintaining your desired weight is a healthy combination of the two, a healthy whole-food, plant-based diet and a healthy regime of exercise. It doesn't have to be running; it can and must be an exercise that you are passionate about, something that you will never get bored doing, something that you don't feel obliged or stressed to do it.

It needs to be a hobby. Otherwise, it won't work. I was always in love with running, and I will always be. Every time I run, I feel free and relaxed, I am in my kingdom, and nobody can touch me.

My advice: Find that sport which makes you feel good about yourself and at the same time makes you burn some calories. I mean playing chess is good, but it won't burn that fat on your belly, right?

You can play ping pong, tennis, basketball, volleyball; you can ski, run, of course, or the simplest of all, walk; power walk, cycle, swim. The list of high-activity sports, either team ones or not, are endless. Find the one you love and combine it with a healthy vegetarian diet, and you are set for life. All the rest is patience and willingness to experiment, and you are on the right path to permanent weight loss.

Now if I have convinced you to adopt a plant-based diet and also to find a sport that you love to do, then it's only a matter of applying them, and I am sure you will see results in the long run. Forget about "fast and easy"; adopt the "gradual and adventurous"!

A Few Things That Will Help You

Here are a few things that will assist you with this adventure you are about to embark on:

Keep a food diary or log. There are some food diaries out there that you can use on your computer, your tablet, mobile phone, or if you are old-fashioned like my ex-wife, you can use a notebook.

Personally, I use two resources. The first is a web page, www.cronometer.com. I log my food there, and it shows me everything, from how many calories I eat and burn to how many carbs, protein, fat, and vitamins I get! You can also program it to tell you how many calories you need to eat to lose weight or gain weight. It's very simple to use, and you can register for free.

The other is an application I use that is developed by the good Doc, Michael Greger, MD, from www.nutritionfacts.org, which is more friendly and simpler. You just note the categories of food you have per serving, and it tells you how healthy your daily consumption is. You can search it on Play Store (for Android) as "Daily Dozen," or you can search it on various search engines as "Dr. Greger's Daily Dozen."

Of course, you are free to use these resources for as long as it takes until it becomes a habit, and your knowledge regarding food has reached a point where you no longer need them.

Your best chance is to follow www.nutritionfacts.org. I wish I knew that site three years ago; it cuts a lot of corners nutrition-wise. Other sources I found useful are the books Vegan for Life by Jack Norris and Virginia Messina and Thrive by Brendan Brazier

Aside from the food diary, you should keep a journal for your exercises that will help you track down how many km/miles you cover if you do running or cycling, and also how many calories you burn. Cronometer© can follow both your food intake and exercise regime. Alternatively, you can keep your journal somewhere else. You can create an Excel spreadsheet as I did at the beginning before I discovered the Cronometer© site, or you can use any other program or application that best suits your needs.

As I stated a lot of times in my first book, Thirsty for Health, everyone is unique, and it is up to you to find your ideal program for weight loss. I am just here sharing my story and my experiences with the hope that something I did will help you. There is no way my weight loss program will work for you 100% because we are not the same. You need to structure your program through your personal struggle and experience. Nothing comes to you; you need to work to earn it, and I am sure of one thing: You must work for your health because it is the only thing that matters.

When I decided to follow a plant-based program, I was already convinced that a vegan way of life would give me healthier options, regarding weight loss, and better running performance.

First-year lesson

The year that I first adopted the plant-based diet and lifestyle was 2013. I was always tired, lethargic, and my running performances had dropped. I was on the verge of eating meat again. What stopped me was a detailed review of my diary from the Cronometer© site, which showed me flat in my face that I required 3000 calories daily because that time I was training for a marathon, whereas I was only getting 2200 calories!!! No wonder I was feeling tired all the time.

After I had found out about that, I increased my calorific intake, and I started to feel better. I started improving my running performance, making it even better than when I was an omnivore. Also, my weight went down, and my fat was replaced with firm muscle mass.

To achieve eating 3000 calories every day, I had a kitchen scale at home where I would measure and weigh everything for a month, and then I would catalog them on the Cronometer©. I did that for a month, and after that, I would rarely scale something except when there was something new, and I didn't know its caloric density.

For example, I knew that if I ate three medium bananas weighing about 80 grams each, I would be getting around 180 calories or the fact that two medium-sized apples give approximately 150 calories.

You will get to this level of knowledge as time progresses, but for a lot of people counting calories, it is very stressful; they want food to be an enjoyment and not a chore.

Count calories

I agree completely with that, but if you want to lose weight, there is a basic, very simple mathematical rule you must follow. You must make sure the calories you consume are less than the calories you burn. If you eat more calories than you can burn, well, guess what happens?... Yes, you guessed right, you GAIN weight.

How else are you going to know that you burn more calories than the ones you consume if you don't count them at least for a month? HOW?

I am sorry, but there is no other way. Even if you go 100% vegan, you still have your plant-based oils, like olive oil, a tablespoon of which has 120 calories! I would have to run a mile to burn 100 to 120 calories! How many of you drown your salad in olive oil, well, those who even eat salads, anyway?

Other sources include nuts, almonds, hazelnuts, and so on. Their fat is exquisite for you, but if you overeat them, then you are adding fat to your already existing fat deposits. Avocados also have a lot of fat.

The primary key is for the calories you take to be less than what your body can burn either by itself or by exercise, and I will explain what I mean by this later.
There are different kinds of calories, and your diet should ideally follow the pattern of 80/10/10, which means your calories should come from carbohydrates by 80%, from protein by 10%, and from fat by 10%.

Now there are many kinds of fat. One of them is the saturated fat, which you want to avoid as much as possible, as dozens of clinical trials and research has shown it is bad for your health. Saturated fat is mostly found in animal foods, such as milk, cheese, and meat. Poultry and fish have less saturated fat than red meat.

The other big category is the unsaturated fat, which is further divided into:

Monounsaturated fat:
Polyunsaturated fat:
Omega-3 fatty acids
Omega-6 fatty acids

These are better for you and are mostly found in plants. Try to limit your intake to 10% of your total calorie intake.

Now, not all nutrients have the same calorie value. For example, one gram of protein and one gram of carbohydrates contain four calories, but one gram of fat contains nine calories! Now you see why you should restrict your intake of fat to 10% and not 30% as many diets claim out there.

You Can't Cheat Evolution.

We evolved over time, living in conditions where our next meal could be weeks apart, and the only thing that kept us alive was our body's ability to store fat and utilize it when we didn't have food to eat for days.

This primordial function did not change; our brain doesn't know that there is a McDonald's or a KFC at every corner of this planet. Food now is no longer a struggle, but every time you sit down for a meal, your brain is telling you to eat like there is no tomorrow because it doesn't know that tomorrow you will eat again!

There is a beautiful book that explains the addiction of modern people to junk food, entitled
Why Humans Like Junk Food by Steven A. Witherly, Ph.D. It blew my mind when I first read it.

Another great book that explains how we evolved—thus will help you to understand a little bit more about how the human body works—is entitled The Fast-5 Diet and the Fast-5 Lifestyle by Bert W. Herring, M.D.

As you can see, I am providing you with books authored by doctors and researchers, not articles online without an indication of a writer or credibility or even a source of information acquired!!!

An example

So let's say you want to eat ten grams of almonds. You will find that they give almost fifty-eight calories. Of those calories, forty-five are fat! About four of them are carbs, and the rest, about nine calories, is protein.

Now you see why you should be careful with dry nuts? Because a big chunk of those forty-five calories will go straight to your fat deposits. You need to satisfy the 80-10-10 rule with a real daily deficit of about 250 to 500 calories for you to see some healthy weight loss results.

By reducing your fat intake and at the same time exercising regularly (running, cycling) more than 30 minutes at a time, your body starts to use your fat as fuel.

If you are thinking, "Oh, Andreas, I can't run more than five minutes, and you talk about running more than thirty minutes," well, I never said it was going to be easy, did I? I said it would be gradual and adventurous.

Best Fat Burning Exercise

The best exercise to lose fat and burn fat is running. I suggest that you should initially start walking, then as you progress with walking, add running intervals, until you stop walking and keep only running. That's your best bet to start putting that overweight body of yours in shape along with a plant-based diet, but if you can't go 100% plant-based, at least try to minimize the animal fat from your diet.

You can also check out my book "How to Train and Finish Your First 5k Race" where there are more detailed instructions on how to incorporate walking and running into your life.

Aside from animal fat, you should also try to limit junk food and processed sugary food. Prefer to eat two apples instead of an apple pie made out of white sugar. Choose to have two bananas frozen and blended into an ice cream instead of eating an ice cream made out of cow's milk, which is full of saturated fat and cholesterol.

Do you see the pattern here? Try and replace the meat you eat with vegan substitutes.You can find pretty much everything as far as meat replacement is concerned or other healthy alternatives, especially if you live in the U.S.A.

Here in Cyprus, you are telling the grocery shop employees you are vegetarian (they don't even know what vegan is) and they look at you like you are a purple alien with three heads!!!

Search the internet to find dietitians and nutritionists or MD's and other doctors that are vegan themselves and advocate a plant-based diet.

Plant-Based Docs

I am going to give you a list of doctors that I have been following since 2013 who helped me immensely with every bit of doubt or question I had about weight loss and exercises and generally if plant-based diets are suitable for humans.
Neal Barnard, M.D.
Web sites: http://www.nealbarnard.org and Physician's Committee for Responsible Medicine (PCRM)

Colin Campbell, M.D.
Website: T. Colin Campbell Center for Nutrition Studies
http://nutritionstudies.org
Caldwell Esselstyn, M.D.
Website: http://www.dresselstyn.com
Joel Fuhrman, M.D.
Website: http://www.drfuhrman.com
Michael Greger, M.D.
Websites: http://www.veganmd.org and NutritionFacts.org
Michael Klaper, M.D.
Website: http://doctorklaper.com
John McDougall, M.D.
Website: http://www.drmcdougall.com
Dean Ornish, M.D.
The Websites http://deanornish.com and Preventive Medicine
Research Institute
Jack Norris RD
Website http://jacknorrisrd.com
Virginia Messina
Website www.theveganrd.com

These are the doctors and dietitians I follow, reading their books, watching their lectures on YouTube or reading their articles. There are dozens more out there who can help you the same way.

Practical Example

Let's examine together a step by step procedure that will help you figure out how many calories you should eat to lose weight healthily and safely.

BMI (Body Mass Index)

BMI is a pretty good indicator of where you stand concerning body fat. It is not absolute as I argued in my previous story in this book, but it gives you an excellent general picture of where you are. Below you can see the BMI categories.

BMI Categories:

Underweight = <18.5
Normal weight = 18.5 - 24.9
Overweight = 25 - 29.9
Obesity = BMI of 30 or greater

The ideal or normal range is for your BMI to be between 18.5 and 24.9

Now go and load the following page:
http://www.nhlbi.nih.gov/health/educational/lose_wt/BMI/bmical
lc.htm

Insert your height in inches and your weight in pounds, or if you prefer in centimeters and kilos, click on the Metric tab, enter your height in cm and your weight in kilos, and hit the button "Compute BMI." My BMI is 23.8 which is pretty good as it indicates the normal range.

If you are above 24.9, then you are overweight, and if you are above 30, you are obese with all the possible health issues you might face if you don't do something about it.

There is a difference between you and other people with weight loss problems: you have decided to do something about it. That is why you are reading this book, and that is why you are reading this practical example of mine.

Shall we continue?

The next piece of information you need to find out is your BMR, your Basal Metabolic Rate, which shows the number of calories you burn if you stay in bed all day!!!

Go to this link http://www.bmi-calculator.net/bmr-calculator/ and insert your height, weight, age, and sex. There is also a metric system too, so click the metric tab and add the same information. Then click the button "Calculate BMR," and the result will appear above in a green line.

My BMR is **1643.6 calories.** This is the number of calories I will burn if I just lay on the bed all day.

Any other extra activity I do, either walking, washing the dishes, riding the bus, running, cycling, or sitting in front of the computer typing will require additional calories.

So let's take me, for example, and you can adjust the numbers to match your own. I am doing my Monday. Let's say I want to lose about 12 pounds (5.5 kg) in 12 weeks, which translates into about a pound a week.

Now there are 3500 calories in a pound (0.45 kg), so to lose a pound at the end of the week, we should burn or create an accumulative deficit of 3500 calories per week, that is a 500-calorie deficit per day.

Now let's see how many calories I need to maintain my weight. We have 1643.6 calories plus activities from the time I wake up to the time I go to bed (no funny business in bed).

Using the Cronometer's "Add Exercise" tab, I can find out how many calories I burn doing my routine tasks of the day.

I will give you my daily routine, and then using the Cronometer© (which is programmed to my height, weight, age, and sex), I will show you how many calories I burn, not counting my BMR.

I wake up at five in the morning, then I use the toilet for about ten minutes (10 calories here). Another five minutes of grooming, brushing my teeth, and washing the face (about 5 calories here).

After that, I get dressed, take the bus to work, and I ride the bus for sixty minutes (that's 23 calories). I get to work where I sit in front of a desk typing on the computer for seven hours and thirty minutes (290 calories).

Coming home by bus is 23 calories. On Mondays, I do cycling on a static bike for about forty-five minutes (437 calories), and I might work on the computer for another hour before I got to bed (about 38 calories).

I know this task may sound daunting, but once you register to Cronometer©, you only do it once, and you can save them, so it is only a matter of copying and pasting the information on other days.

After I add all those calories I need to eat, I come to the conclusion that on Monday, I have to eat 2469 calories, let's make them 2500, to maintain my weight. So on Monday, if I want to lose a pound a week as I mentioned before, I need to create a 500-calorie deficit and eat 2000 calories.

I am going to repeat that it may sound daunting, but you only need to make it for a week because this way, you will cover your whole exercise and daily routine.

Let me show you now how easy it is to do the same for Tuesday.

All the daily tasks are the same nothing changes. The only thing that changes is that on Tuesday, I go and do my track repetitions. That means I only need to calculate those I have programmed to do (5 repeats x 800 meters).

I go to Cronometer©, type "track," choose "track practice," and I input the minutes this exercise will take me. So I know it's going to take about forty-five minutes, which translates into about 525 calories.

So now I have my BMR of 1643, plus 389 (my daily routine, minus the cycling), plus my track running, which accumulate to 2557 calories, let's say 2600. So on Tuesday, I need to eat 2100 calories to be okay with the 500-calorie deficit a day program (substantially, burn more than you eat, that is).

I think you got the algorithm and the philosophy of what you need to do. If you don't want to do this for any reason, you can go to a doctor or a registered dietitian, and he/she can prepare the program for you along with what kind of exercises you must do.

The secret is that you should see this as a life-changing event. It should become a lifestyle and not just a temporary diet. It should become a way of life; that's the only way to lose those pounds and never gain them back. If you don't make it your lifestyle, you will just suffer from a yo-yo weight for the rest of your life, which is very hazardous to your health and your psychological and emotional state of mind.

The Mystery Of B12

The decision.

When I decided to become a plant-based eater, I did not know how difficult it would be for me to get accustomed to the new way that this lifestyle demands of you.

Don't think for a second that a plant-based diet is just another "diet" people follow to lose some weight and then return to their old habits.

If you want to see results with a plant-based diet, you need to understand that it is not just a diet; it is a lifestyle.

One of the first things I learned about following a plant based diet is that I would need to supplement it with vitamin B12 because B12 along with Vitamin D is not found in the plant world. I read that you don't need to start taking it right away but after three years of a plant-based diet because B12 storage in the body can last for an extended period.

I chose to play it safe, so I did take the supplement from the start. I did not look into it. I just use a particular vegan brand, and I am getting a pill with 1000 mcg of B12 daily.

I did that for the first two years, and I was completely satisfied with the supplement. It was quick and easy, and I was not worried about having a B12 deficiency. My latest blood test results last year showed that my B12 levels were at 601 pg/ml, and the reference values are 181 to 900, which means I am ok, and the supplements work just fine.

Search, search, search and when you are done, search again.

I am always a staunch supporter of using as little pills as possible even if they are supplements. Don't trust doctors too much. Don't get me wrong, I am not against western medicine as many people are. I just take the good things out of it, like diagnostic exams, such as the Pap smear, for example, which is a significant western medicine accomplishment as it saves a lot of women from cervical cancer.

On the other hand, western medicine discovered and manufactured chemical drugs to fight cancer. That kind of medicine in most cases kills the patients and not cancer itself.

My philosophy is search, research, and apply your findings; keep what is best for you and repeat the whole process as often as possible and whenever your lifestyle allows you to do it.

So that's what I did. At some point, I wasn't feeling well with myself using a supplement, even if it proved to me that it worked. I didn't have any other serious reason for taking it except that I had read it in a few well-respected and full of resources vegan web pages that advised people to take B12 supplementation.

The fact that I had to take a pill every day was not something that I enjoyed or liked. I placed a personal bet that in 2015 I will figure out a way to completely remove the B12 supplement from my life, my goal was to "supplement the supplement" or at least reduce its daily use.

This article is the journey I took to solve the riddle of the B12 vitamin.

Questions, lots of them.

The first question I asked myself was **"what is vitamin B12, anyway?"** and it turns out it is only found in bacteria, eggs, and—surprise, surprise—in foods that have an animal origin.

Cobalamin, aka B12, does not occur in plants but is synthesized by certain bacteria, fungi, and algae, which constitute the ultimate source of all cobalamin found in nature.

Now does that mean that we should eat meat? No! Then again, I am not of those "vegan" activists that claim that the natural food of humans is only plant-based. We evolved eating some meat as a species; archeological evidence supports this.

I am just a plant-based eater because I found it to be healthier for me, for the animals (they don't get slaughtered), and for the planet (it's not systematically destroyed)—and for one last reason: because I freaking can.

I **can** be a plant-based eater because the supplement technology allows it, plain and straightforward!

Next question I asked myself was **"why do we need B12, anyway?"** Why do we have to take this particular vitamin?

Well, being the little researcher I am—as you can figure out from my first book "Thirsty For Health"—I started looking and reading articles online, scientific research papers and documents; also videos and books. In a nutshell, Vitamin B12 is essential for our health since it is responsible for proper red blood cell formation and the development of the nervous system.

So, basically, if you want to have blood running in your veins and remember what you did five seconds ago, you need this nutrient!

Also, studies have shown that a cause-and-effect relationship has been established between the dietary intake of vitamin B12 and

- The contribution to normal neurological and psychological functions.
- The contribution to normal homocysteine metabolism.
- The reduction of tiredness and fatigue.

My next question was **"how long can I last without taking any B12 at all?"** It turns out that the answer to this depends on the stored B12 you have in your body and keep in mind that our body is not always 100% healthy. The liver also stores extra B12, and our body does have a recycling process of the vitamin. The bacteria in our colon make vitamin B12. However, the absorption of B12 takes place higher up in the gastrointestinal tract, near the end of the small intestine.

I concluded that it would take an adult that completely ceased to consume B12 three to ten years to develop a deficiency. This incredible machine that accommodates our soul, the human body, typically stores about 1 to 3 mg of vitamin B12.

Usually, if no supplementation occurs and no animal products are eaten, 1 mg of stored vitamin B12 would last for three years, 2 mg for five years and 3 mg for six years if the body has no health issues. The mentioned periods drop to 2, 3.6, and 4 years respectively if there are absorption problems.

The next logical question was **"What are the possible reasons for the vitamin B12 malabsorption?"**

Memory lane.

When I was a student in Greece, I was a heavy smoker, a heavy drinker of soda and coffee, a big consumer of fast junk food, and an excessive meat eater. All this poor nutrition got its toll on my digestive system, and years later, I was diagnosed with stomach ulcer and also duodenum ulcer. You can find more in my book "Thirsty for Health," my journey towards finding my health and, as a result, my happiness.

When I had my first stomach inspection at the age of 31, the doctor said that I had old ulcers or ulcers that were healed. That means that from the age of 20 until 31, I was killing myself internally, eating basically what most people eat in the so-called western societies, which was meat, dairy products, and lots of processed food. That is why I had repeated ulcers in my stomach.

I remember that I was suffering from depression when I was a student, and I didn't know why, but now, after learning about B12 deficiency, I can see there is substantial evidence that maybe I had been B12 deficient.

The concentration suggested for defining vitamin B12 deficiency, based on metabolic indicators, is: < 150 pmol/L (203 pg/mL) for plasma vitamin B12.

Deficiency...

There are mainly two reasons why a person doesn't get enough B12: a) reduced dietary intake and b) lack of absorption because of medical problems.

Some medical conditions that prevent the absorption of the vitamin are gastric atrophy, pernicious anemia, fish tapeworm infection, bacterial overgrowth in the upper intestine, various medications like Proton pump inhibitors, and much more.

The cause of my ulcer except for the bad food I was consuming for many years was also an infection by Helicobacter Pylori which probably resulted in gastric atrophy, which is one of the reasons for severe cobalamin (B12) malabsorption.

Maybe that explains the depression and insomnia, mood swings, and lack of concentration and attention I was suffering from. The new information I found out about B12 deficiency was a real eye-opener.

People with gastric problems usually have decreased stomach acid secretion and also a drop in the digestive enzyme, pepsin, that results in a diminished digestion of vitamin B12 from protein, inhibiting some B12 to be available for absorption.

Some reasons for B12 poor absorption are:

- Low dietary intake
- Veganism
- Lacto-Ovo vegetarianism
- Low animal-sourced food intake
- Inadequate stores and intake by breastfed infants
- Malabsorption
- Gastric atrophy and malabsorption (from food)
- Pernicious anemia
- Ileal disease
- Chronic pancreatitis
- Parasitic infections
- Medications

In the list above, they don't include omnivores because they eat adequate quantities of meat; thus, they are not considered to have a B12 deficiency.

A hypothesis for you.

Herbivorous animals, like sheep and cows, eat grass. Now the grass gets cobalt from the ground. Cobalt is used by microorganisms within the rumen (2nd stomach) to make Vitamin B12. Vitamin B12 is then absorbed in the small intestine and transported throughout the body by the blood, with excess being stored in the liver. Then, the humans slaughter the sheep and cows and take the vitamin B12 through the meat.

My question is this, "when was the last time you ate a lamb or a cow that had eaten grass from pasture?" The answer is "very rarely." Most animals these days are raised in CAFOs (Concentrated Animal Feeding Operations), the new prisons for animals to be raised and slaughtered as I describe in my book "Thirsty For Health."

There—trust me—the animals do not eat grass; they are fed soy beans, corn, and any other thing you can imagine except for their natural food.
For me, the fact that omnivores are not in the B12 deficiency alert list is wrong.
Dairy products do not have enough B12, and about the meat, we don't know if the animals created the vitamin in the first place because of the lack of grass (and consequently cobalt) from their diet.

My advice is that no matter your diet, you should check your B12. You have nothing to lose and everything to gain; at least you will be able to sleep easy at night knowing that your cells are divided as they should, and you have top enzymatic reactions, proper metabolism of carbohydrates and fatty acids, and a healthy nervous system.
Some test methods that you can use to define B12 deficiency are:

Mean cell volume and blood film examination
- Serum Cobalamin
- Plasma Total Homocysteine (tHcy)

- Plasma Methylmalonic Acid (MMA)
- Holotranscobalamin
- Bone marrow examination

My journey on finding out if I could discover alternative ways of getting B12 was a complete success because I learned so many things that enabled me to understand and utilize this vitamin better.

Fortified foods like some of the many different brands of breakfast cereals out there is a good daily source of B12 and also nutritional yeast.

I use it on my spaghetti, in my smoothies, on my popcorn, in soups, everywhere I find it handy, so that's an extra source of B12 getting into my body.

The internal functions.

Now let's have some mathematics. Our body can only absorb 1.5 to 2 mcg of B12 at a time, and our receptors of B12 need about 4 to 6 hours to unload their cargo. So it's a good tactic to get some B12, either from a supplement or from food, every 6 hours.

The other thing you can do is to take 2500 mcg once a week, and that will give you about 3.5 mcg a day, 3000 mcg weekly will give you 4.2 mcg a day, and 5000 mcg will give you 7 mcg a day.

Any more than 7 mcg a day will do nothing as the body can't absorb more, and you'll end up peeing the excess B12.

It is better to get between 4 to 7 mcg a day than the 2.4 mcg that is recommended; that number was based on some fragile research years ago. Recent studies suggest 4 to 7 mcg a day. Either chewable, sublingual or liquid supplement is fine, and it will work. However, there are researchers out there that highly recommend the use of sublingual supplement because of its better absorption. Also, always consult your doctor about issues like dosage and other related topics.

My tactic.

What I do now varies depending on whether I am training for a marathon or not; if I am, I will take a supplement of 100 mcg daily and a 1000-mcg pill three times a week. If I am not training for a marathon, then I will just stop doing the daily supplement.

The reason I supplement daily is that when I am training, I need more of everything, more protein, carbs, fat, vitamins minerals, and so on.

Math haters turn away. (Wink)

From 100 mcg I get every day, 1.5 to 2 mcg is absorbed by the receptors, and the rest 1% is stored in the body which means, 100 minus 1.5 equals 98.5, divided by 100 equals 0.988 mcg, so I get approximately 2.48 to 2.98 mcg daily. This is fine for the daily recommendation, but I want to reach the "4 to 7 mcg" limit, so I additionally get an extra 3000 mcg a week, which, if we apply the same math and divide by seven, gives me an extra 4.2 daily. And a total of 6.68 to 7.18 mcg.

Plus, I am getting B12 from nutritional yeast and other fortified foods.

Well, that's my story as far as the controversial vitamin B12 is concerned. I hope I helped some of you.

Conclusion

I won't take any more of your time, I hope you enjoyed the book, and I hope I helped you in some way. To recap, the recipe for a successful, healthy weight loss without gaining it back is a balanced combination of a plant-based diet/lifestyle and exercise.

My advice is that you should at some point adopt a 100% plant-based diet, but even if this is out of the scope of your goals, you can at least try to adopt a lifestyle that is 80% plant-based and 20% animal-based; it is in your health's best interest.

Try to limit your fat to 10% of your total calories and always consult a physician, a doctor or a dietitian before embarking on and during a weight loss program.

Here I told my story and also gave some advice for the things that worked for me, but you should always consult a doctor or a trained medical professional before making any dramatic changes that may have an adverse impact on your health.

In case you are a physician or a scientist in the health area and see something that is not correct in my book, I urge you to point it out, and I will gladly do my very best to fix it.

My warmest regards,

Andreas Michaelides

Other books by Andreas Michaelides

Thirsty For Health

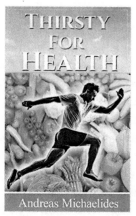

A truly eye-opening book that should and will make your question yourself and everything you have done so far diet and lifestyle wise. Obesity, caffeine and junk food addiction, smoking and digestive problems? This is the place you can start answering your most asked questions. A book you wish you had found earlier, an amazing story that had to be told to help others not to go through the same misery. In these pages, you will learn how to regain control over your life, how to find strength from within to go through life's numerous challenges, successfully overcome addictions and finally tune into genuine health and happiness. You are the alchemist, the architect of your life and no one else but you have the power to make the change. Be the change that you want to see in the world. You can start now, and this book will help you do that and more, and you will also learn how to live long and live well.

The Food I Grew Up With...Veganized!

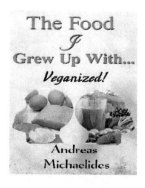

I wrote this book first to thank my mother for never letting me without food on the table and secondly to show to people out there that they can thrive on a plant-based diet. The most important of all they don't have to start from zero as food is concerned I hope I will show with this book that you can transform many of your old food into new versions of plant based ones. This book is not a cookbook although it contains a lot of the food recipes I used to and still eating today. All the recipes are a result of many interviews with

47

my mother which without her this book would never be possible. This book basically shows one aspect of my psyche as food is concerned and how I deal with it transitioning from an omnivore to a herbivore.

How to train and finish your first 5k race.

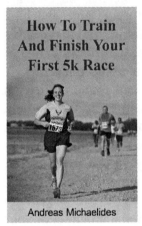

How To Train And Finish Your First 5k Race

Andreas Michaelides

You can watch other people running on the TV, playing football, basketball, or baseball. At least those guys are getting paid to run and jump and tackle. Why should you go through this torture of actually getting up from your soft chair and making yourself go through this ordeal? Why would you enter this nightmare? Why not continue your ignorant bliss of a lovely sedentary life where all you need to do is push the buttons of a remote control, and then people in the box can live your desires, your fantasies, your dreams, and ultimately, your life?

Please write a review.

I consider myself as a person that wants to think that I am constantly improving my books, my work and myself. I am always trying to deliver to my readers the best quality and current information out there as my area of interest and expertise is a concern which is Health, Nutrition, and Exercise.

To accomplish that I need feedback from you and the only feedback I know that will help me achieve a relative perfection in all areas of my life is your valuable reviews, so I know where I am wrong or where I have made mistakes and errors.

There is no such thing as a perfect book out there, perfection for one person is a sloppy work for other, so to satisfy as much as people out there my books need to be regularly updated and it doesn't matter if it's in electronic form (Kindle) or paperback form.

If you found this book useful, please leave your review with all your thoughts, don't hold back, it will only take a few minutes of your time.

If you didn't like this book, please let me know by contacting me, and I will give my best shot to fix the issue.

Thank you very much,

My warmest regards

Andreas Michaelides

Sources

Links

http://www.webmd.com/diet/guide/types-of-fats-topic-overview?page=1
http://www.nhlbi.nih.gov/health/educational/lose_wt/BMI/bmicalc.htm
www.muscleandstrength.com/articles/body-types-ectomorph-mesomorph-endomorph.html
www.britannica.com/EBchecked/topic/178685/ectomorph
www.bodybuilding.com/fun/best_ectomorph_workout.htm
www.cbc.ca/news/technology/thin-people-may-be-fat-on-the-inside-doctors-warn-1.681897
www.lef.org/Magazine/2015/2/The-Deadly-Consequences-Of-Excess-Abdominal-Fat/Page-01?p=1
www.health.harvard.edu/staying-healthy/abdominal-fat-and-what-to-do-about-it
www.scientificamerican.com/article/why-does-fat-deposit-on-t
www.cbass.com/Deepfatdeadly.htm
www.patient.co.uk/health/obesity-and-overweight-in-adults
www.mentalhelp.net/poc/view_doc.php?type=doc&id=5914&cn=219
www.cdc.gov/healthyweight/assessing/bmi
www.cdc.gov/healthyweight/assessing/bmi/adult_bmi
www.nlm.nih.gov/medlineplus/ency/article/007196.htm
www.nhlbi.nih.gov/health/educational/lose_wt/bmitools.htm
www.webmd.com/men/weight-loss-bmi
www.bodybuildingpro.com/bodytypeinformation.html
www.bodybuilding.com/fun/becker3.htm
www.muscleandstrength.com/articles/body-types-ectomorph-mesomorph-endomorph.html
www.directlyfitness.com/store/3-body-types-explained-ectomorph-mesomorph-endomorph
http://www.pcrm.org/health/saturated-fat

Publications

1.   Chapter 8
Overweight and obesity (high body mass index)
W. Philip T. James, Rachel Jackson-Leach,
Cliona Ni Mhurchu, Eleni Kalamara,
Maryam Shayeghi, Neville J. Rigby,
Chizuru Nishida and Anthony Rodgers

2.   The space of human body shapes: reconstruction and parameterization from range scans
Brett Allen Brian Curless Zoran Popovi´c
University of Washington

3.   Body Mass Index (BMI)
What Does It Mean to Have a High BMI?

4.   Centers for Disease Control and Prevention National Center for Chronic Disease Prevention and Health Promotion Division of Population Health
Body Mass Index Measurement in Schools

5.   Department of Health and Human Services
Centers for Disease Control and Prevention
 Body Mass Index: Considerations for Practitioners

6.   BODY   TYPES   (Description,   Training,   Diet)
How Can One Overcome Genetic Disadvantages?

7.   Body Composition, Body Fatness

8.   CONSTRUCTION OF THE BODY MASS INDEX-FOR-AGE STANDARDS
6.1 Indicator-specific methodology

9.   National Obesity Observatory – Body Mass Index as a measure of obesity June 2009

10.   NIH Publication No. 06-5830 June 2006 – Facts About Healthy Weight

11.   Body Mass Index and Health
A Publication of the USDA Center for Nutrition Policy and Promotion, March 2000

12.   Statistical Brief #247: Trends in Health Care Expenditures by Body Mass Index (BMI) Category for Adults in the U.S. Civilian Noninstitutionalized Population, 2001 and 2006 – Medical Expenditure Panel Survey, Agency for Healthcare Research and Quality.

13.   NIH Publication No. 04–4158Updated October 2012

CPSIA information can be obtained
at www.ICGtesting.com
Printed in the USA
LVOW07s2026101017

551899LV00015B/1572/P